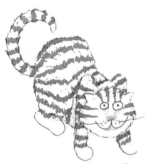

Test Your Cat's M...

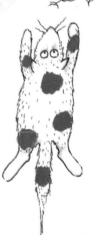

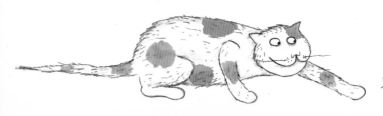

Test Your Cat's Mental Health

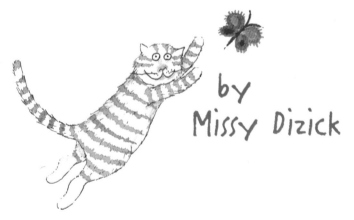

by
Missy Dizick

Adams Media Corporation
Holbrook, Massachusetts

Published by Adams Media Corporation
260 Center Street, Holbrook, MA 02343

ISBN: 1-55850-712-4

Printed in Korea

J I H G F E D C B A

Library of Congress Cataloging-in-Publication Data
Test your cat's mental health / Missy Dizick.
    p.   cm.
ISBN 1-55850-712-4 (pbk.)
1. Cats—Humor. I. Title.
PN6231.C23D59   1997
741.5973—dc21   96-54733
                                  CIP

This book is available at quantity discounts
for bulk purchases. For information,
call 1-800-872-5627 (in Massachusetts, 617-767-8100).

Visit our home page at http://www.adamsmedia.com

To my husband Ron, who, before moi, had no idea how great it is to share your life with a mess of cats. Now he knows. Many thanks for his unwavering support and many suggestions. Especially, thanks for the hilarious Kitty Weirdness Scale, which he wrote as his real—life self, Dr. Ron McKinney, Ph.D. Without the input of a real psychologist, it might have been totally silly.

Thanks also to my editor Laura Morin for her great feedback, and to my agent Loretta Barrett for the obvious reasons.

INTRODUCTION

Does your cat drool and stare into space? Moon you at the breakfast table? Do you sometimes find him halfway up the drapes, or doing the backstroke across the kitchen floor with a sprig of catnip up his nose? Probably so, since all cats are weird, which is one of the reasons we love them.

But how weird is your cat? Lovably eccentric, normally weird, or off the scale? You may have wondered at times, but now you can find out for sure. Just take this fun and easy test, and add up the points. This will give you your cat's score on the KWS, or Kitty Weirdness Scale. Then consult the handy scoring guide at the back of the book, and you will know whether or not your cat needs professional help.

ATTITUDE

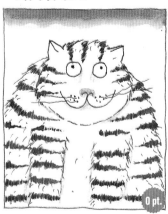

Mellow

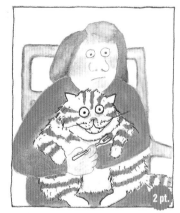

Fair—swaps food for love

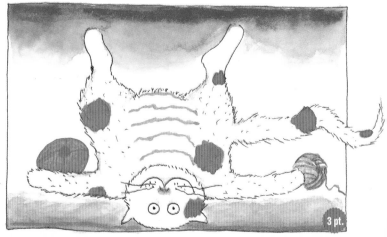

Playful

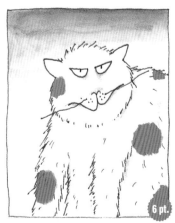

Surly

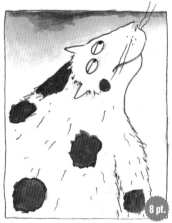

Haughty—thinks self to be
of royal blood

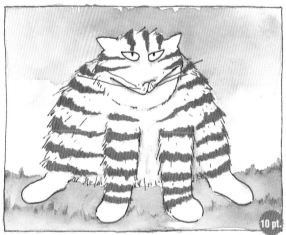

Believes self to be center of the universe

BARFING

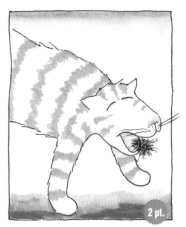

Hairball

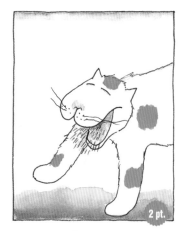

Grass

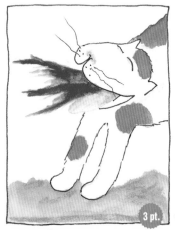

Grasshopper

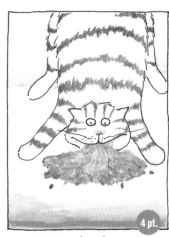

Whole Feeding

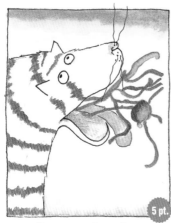

Prey—guts only

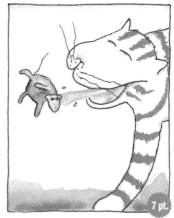

Prey—entire

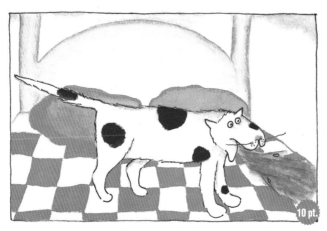

On your bed

BEGGING

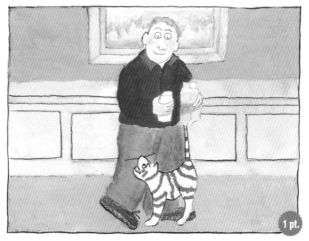

Milk

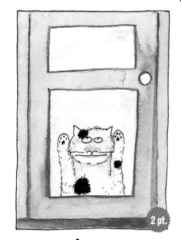

Door

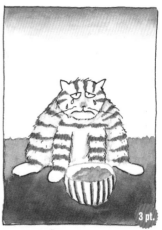

I don't like this kind

1 pt.

2 pt.

3 pt.

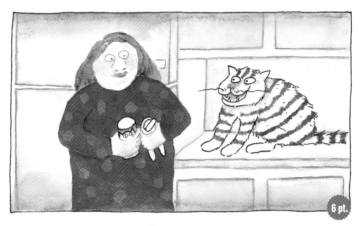

Can opener

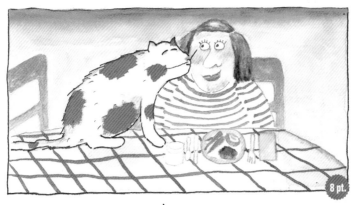

Dinner

BODY LANGUAGE

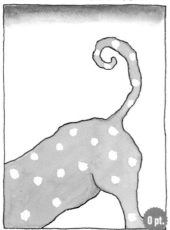

Inquiring tail wants to know

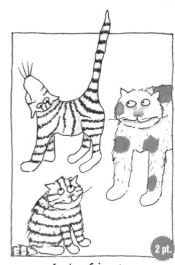

Snubs friends

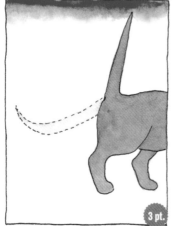

Flips you off

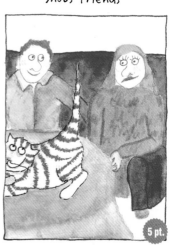

Moons company

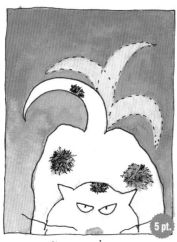

Use caution

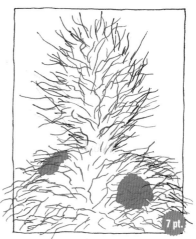

Let's fight

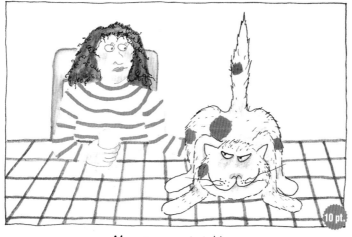

Moons you at table

DESTRUCTION

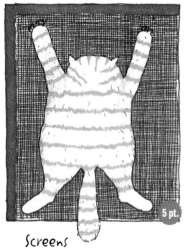

Screens   5 pt.

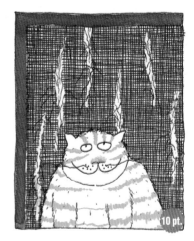

Screens—total devastation   10 pt.

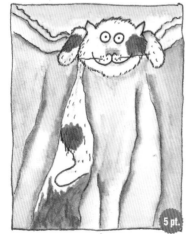

Curtains   5 pt.

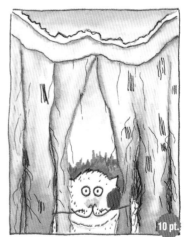

Curtains—total devastation   10 pt.

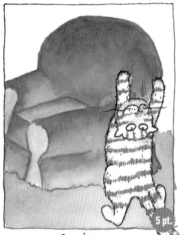

furniture

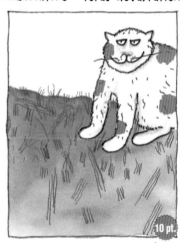

furniture—total devastation

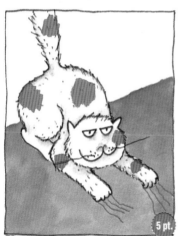

Carpets

Carpets—total devastation

DRINKING

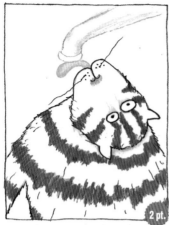

Faucet

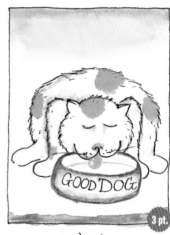

Dog's dish

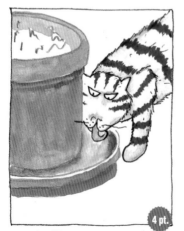

Plant saucer

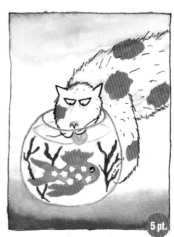

Fishbowl

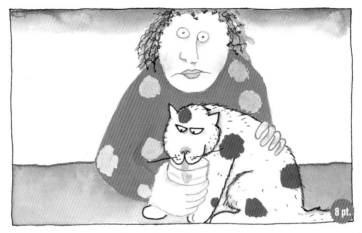

Your glass

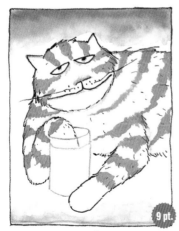

Dunking

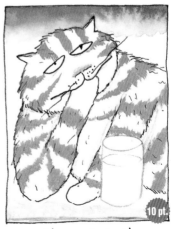

Dunking and slurping

DROOLING

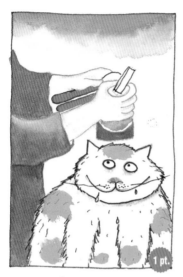

Can opener

1 pt.

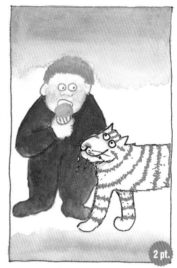

Ice cream

2 pt.

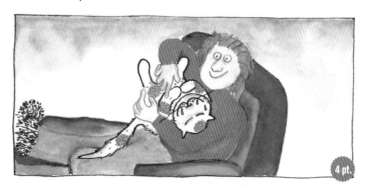

When purring

4 pt.

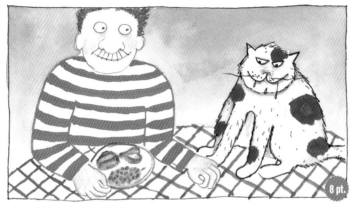

On dinner table

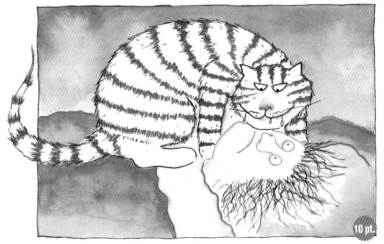

In your face at 4 a.m.

EATING

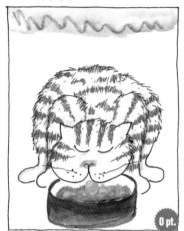

Easy to please

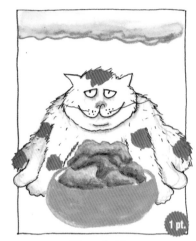

The glutton

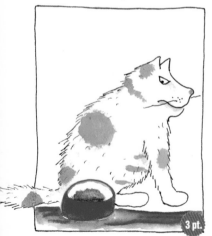

Fussy

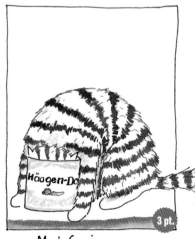

Mad for ice cream

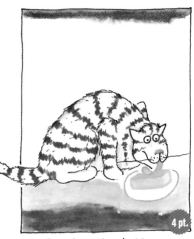

Samples the butter

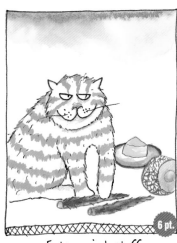

Eats weird stuff

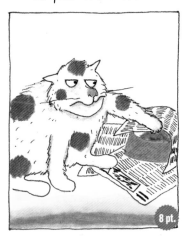

Buries food

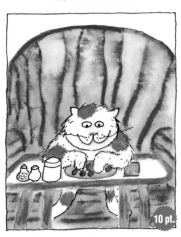

Has own TV tray

EXERCISING

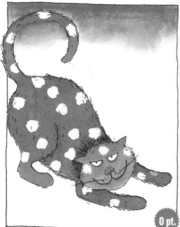

Stretching

0 pt.

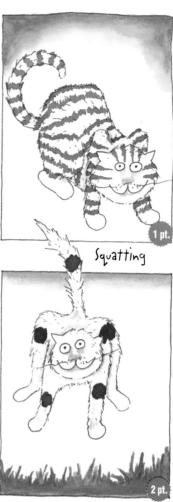

Squatting

1 pt.

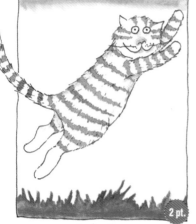

Springing

2 pt.

Leaping

2 pt.

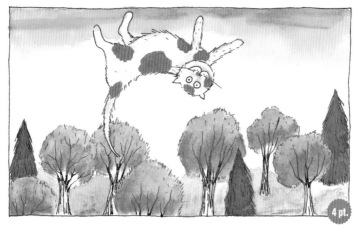

Backflips

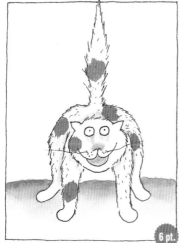

Sticks the landing

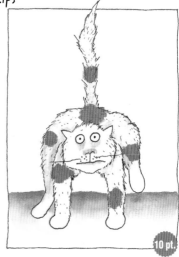

Sticks the landing on one foot

FIGHTING

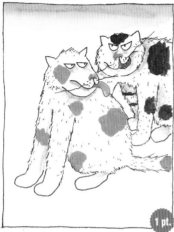

With other cats, minor   1 pt.

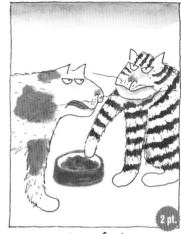

Over food   2 pt.

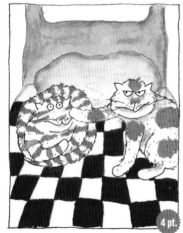

Over best spot on the bed   4 pt.

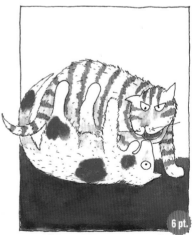

With other cats, major   6 pt.

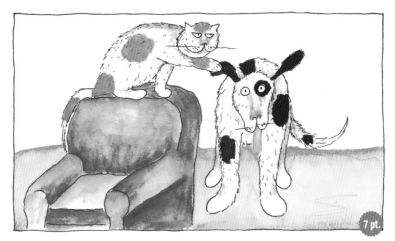

With the right dog

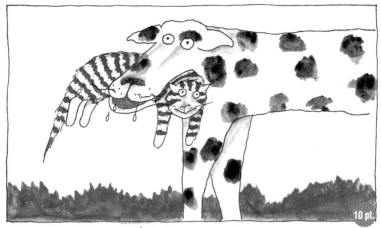

With the wrong dog

IN THE GARDEN

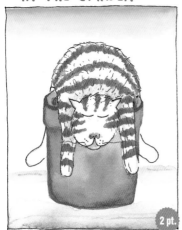

Nap

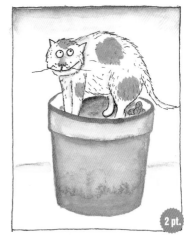

Litter pan

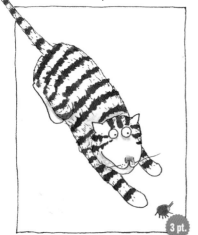

Bugs

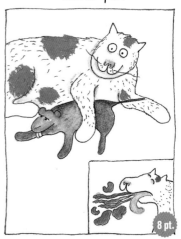

Gophers (greasy grimy gopher guts)

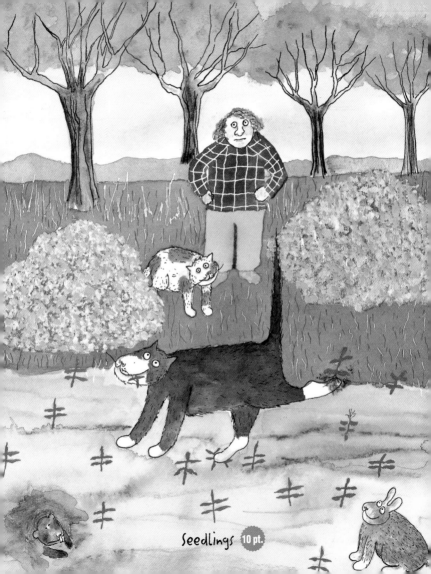

Seedlings 10 pt.

GETTING INTO THINGS

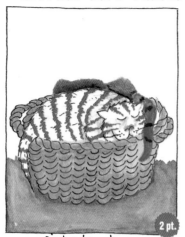

Dirty laundry,
+3 pt. bonus if clean

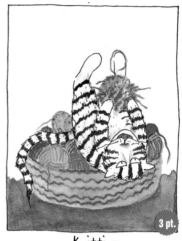

Knitting

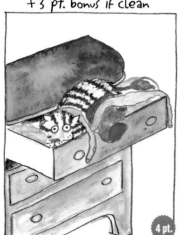

Lingerie

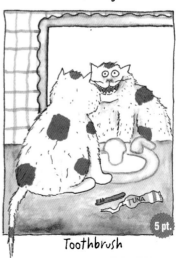

Toothbrush

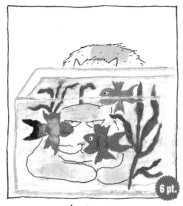

Fishbowl

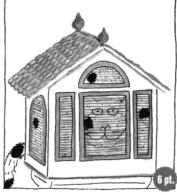

Birdcage

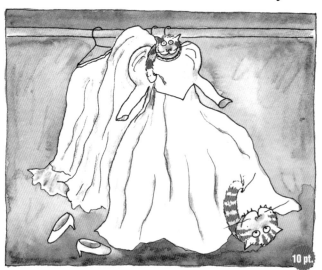

Wedding gown

GETTING STUCK

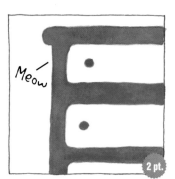

Dresser drawer

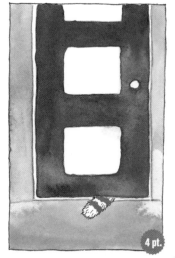

Closet

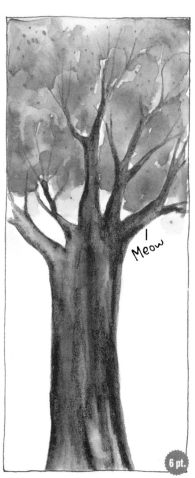

Tree

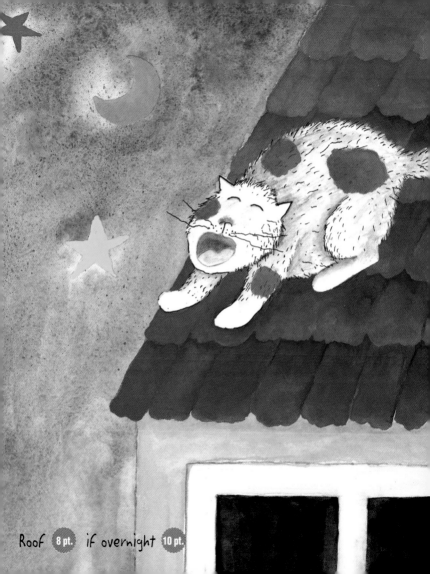

Roof **8 pt.** if overnight **10 pt.**

GOING TO THE VET

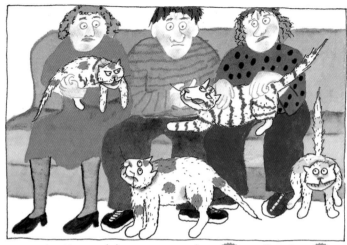

In the waiting room: peeing **2 pt.**   Fighting **5 pt.**

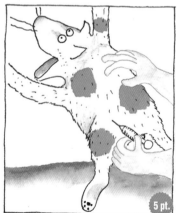

Leaps away from shot **5 pt.**

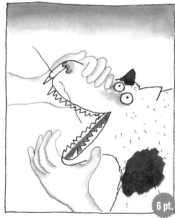

Bites during dental exam **6 pt.**

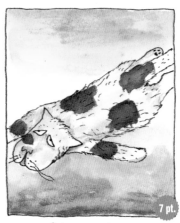

Sick as a dog,
runs up big vet bill

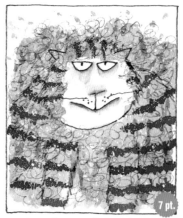

Flea bath—incontinence

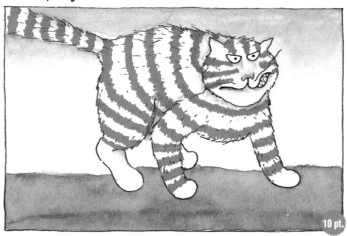

Better now—ungrateful snarl

HIDING

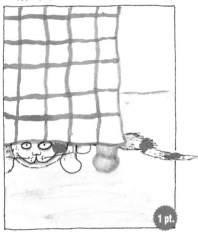

Occasionally

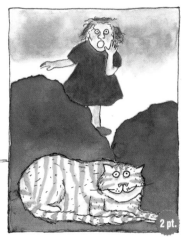

When called

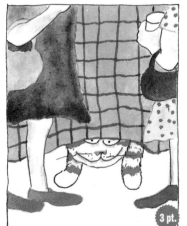

From strangers

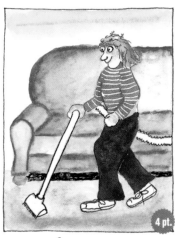

From vacuum

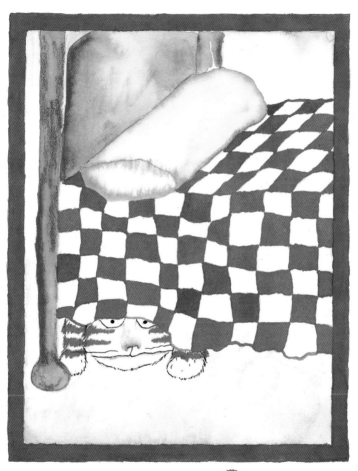

23 hours a day 10 pt.

HUNTING: METHOD

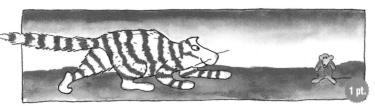

Stalking

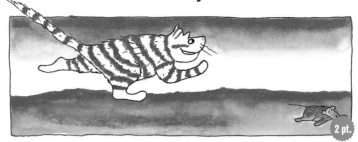

Pouncing

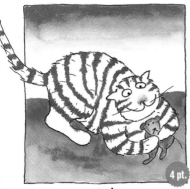

Catching

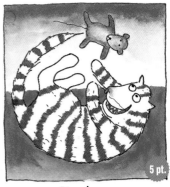

Playing

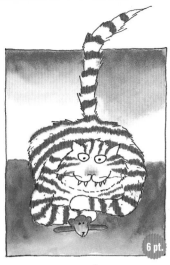

Torturing

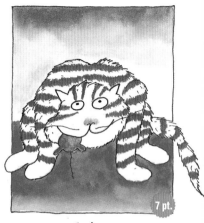

Eating

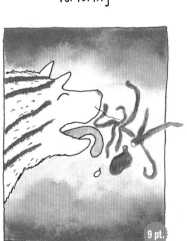

Barfing

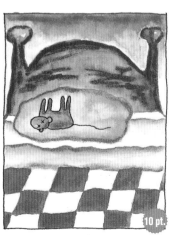

Trophy

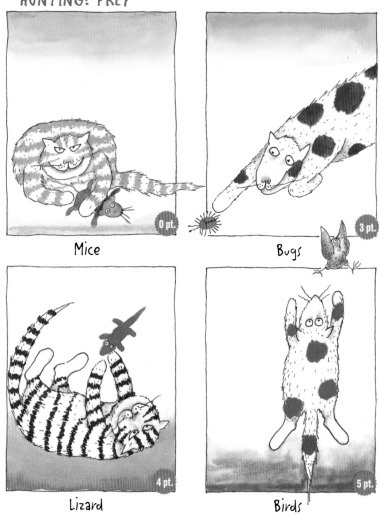

Mice

Bugs

Lizard

Birds

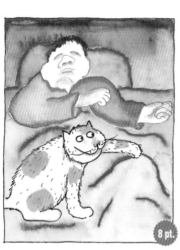

feet under covers

Large dog

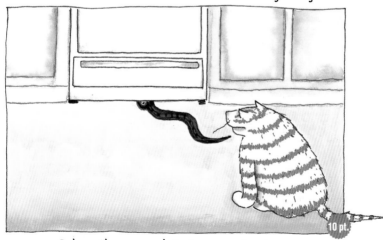

Brings live prey into house and releases

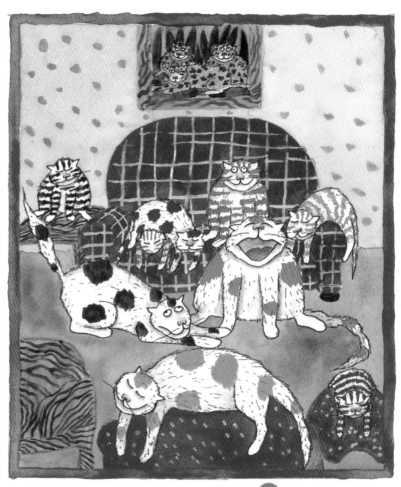

Stretching, yawning **0** pt.

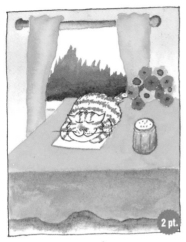

Paperweight

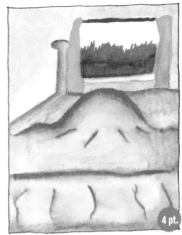

Won't move when bed is made

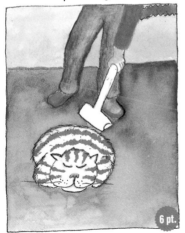

Won't move for vacuum cleaner

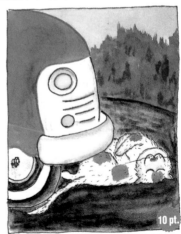

Won't move to save life

MOODS

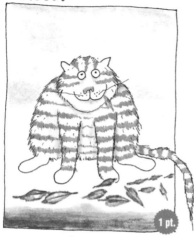

Happy — 1 pt.

Gloomy — 2 pt.

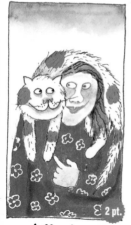

Affectionate — 2 pt.

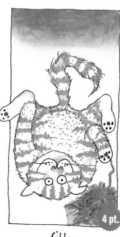

Silly — 4 pt.

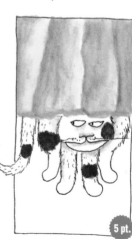

Anxious — 5 pt.

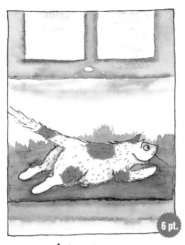

Adventurous 6 pt.

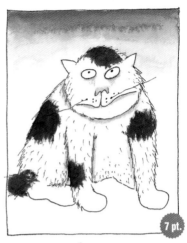

Grumpy 7 pt.

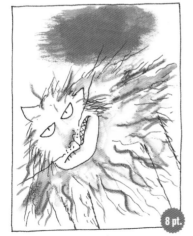

Aggressive 8 pt.

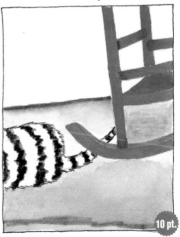

Self-destructive 10 pt.

IN THE NIGHT

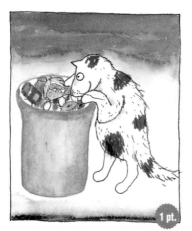

Checks the garbage

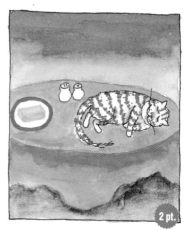

Sleeps on the table

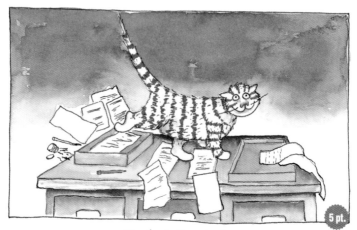

Trashes the desk

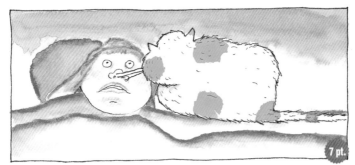

Whiskers in your face

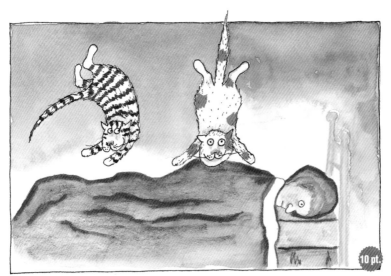

Gymnastics on the bed

PERSONAL CLEANLINESS

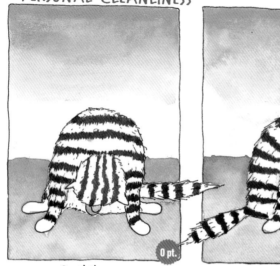

Fastidious — 0 pt.

Excessive — 1 pt.

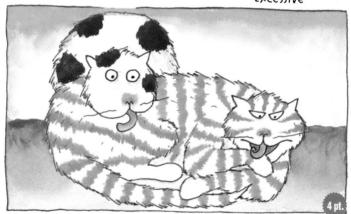

Boundary problems — 4 pt.

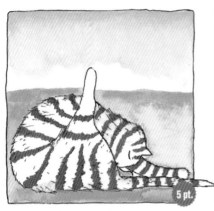

Post-potty

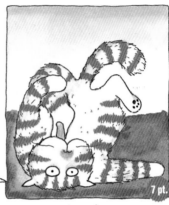

Obsessive

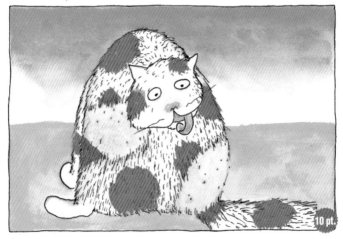

Bald spots

PLAYING: APPARATUS

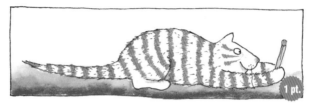

Pencil

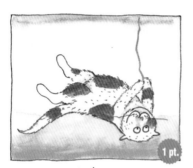

String

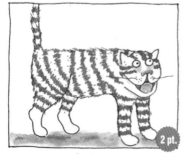

Foil ball

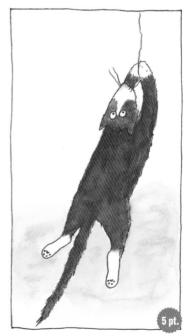

String—airborne

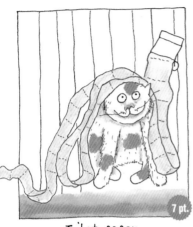

Toilet paper

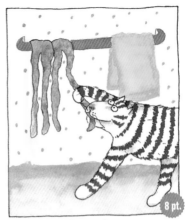

Pantyhose

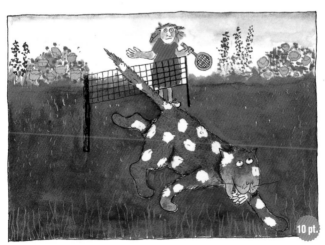

Shuttlecock

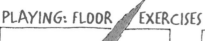
PLAYING: FLOOR EXERCISES

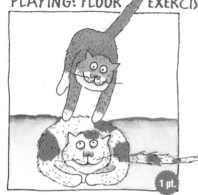

Tackling — 1 pt.

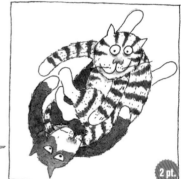

Wrestling — 2 pt.

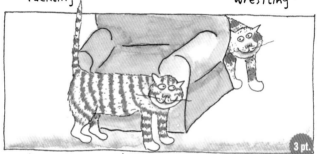

Hide-and-seek — 3 pt.

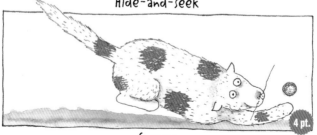

Soccer — 4 pt.

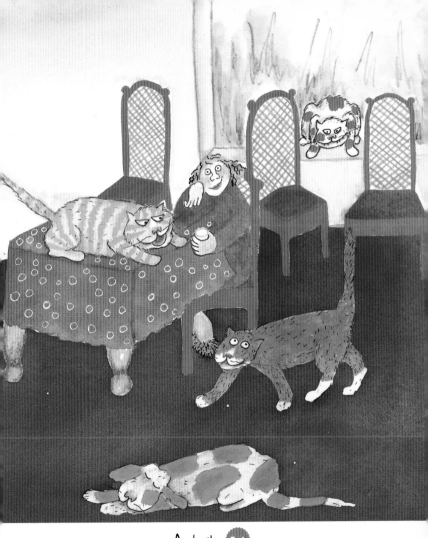

Ambush 5 pt.

ON THE POTTY

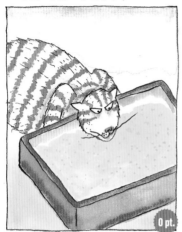

Inspection

0 pt.

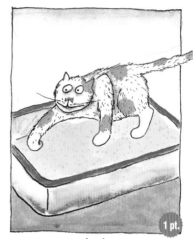

Digging

1 pt.

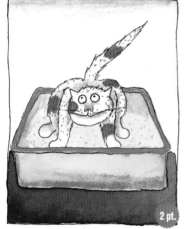

Hits

2 pt.

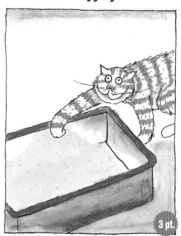

The cover-up

3 pt.

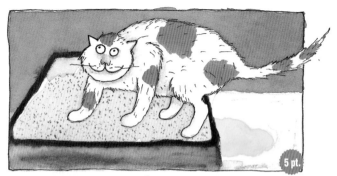

Misses

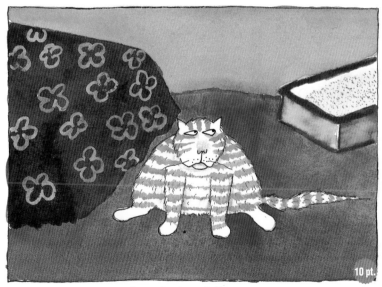

Confuses bed and litter pan

RELATIONSHIPS WITH CHILDREN

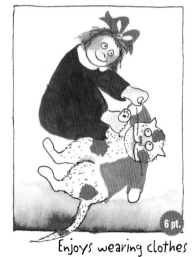

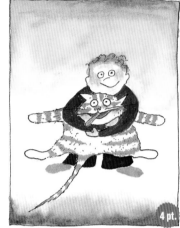

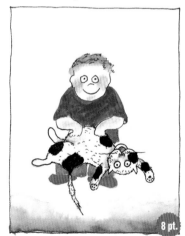

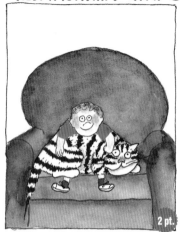

2 pt.

Enjoys sitting with child

4 pt.

Enjoys being carried by child

6 pt.

Enjoys wearing clothes

8 pt.

Enjoys abuse

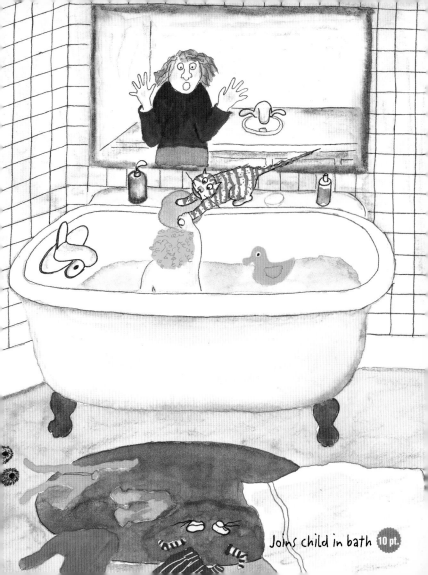

Joins child in bath **10 pt.**

SLEEP HABITS

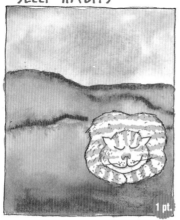

On your feet

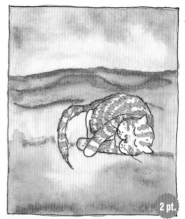

At your back

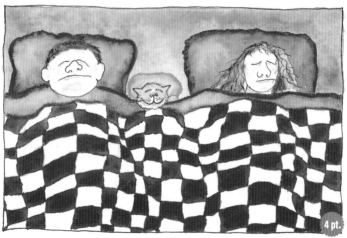

Under the covers

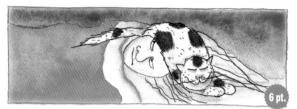

On your head

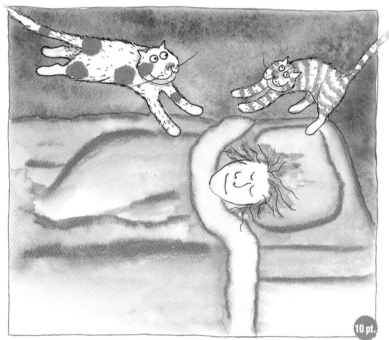

Playing leapfrog

SOCIABILITY

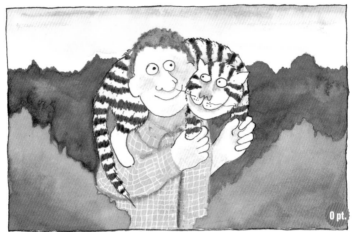

Snuggle bunny

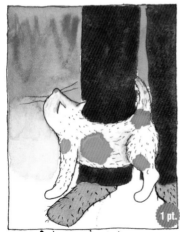

Rubs against leg

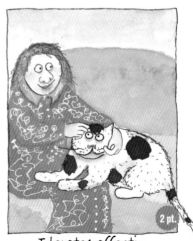

Tolerates affection

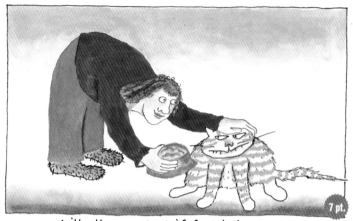

Will allow contact if food is involved

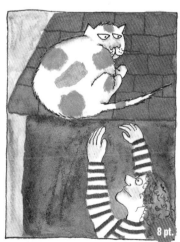

Keep your distance

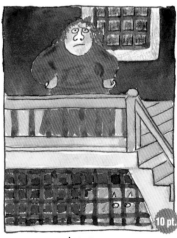

Withdrawn

STAKING TERRITORY

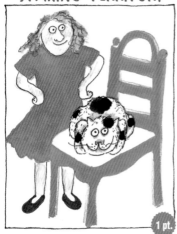

Chair   1 pt.

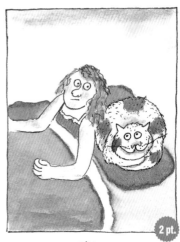

Pillow   2 pt.

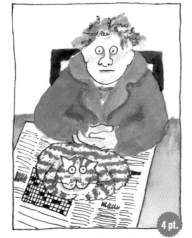

Crossword puzzle   4 pt.

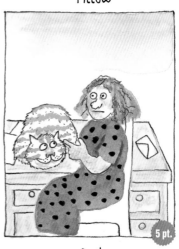

Desk   5 pt.

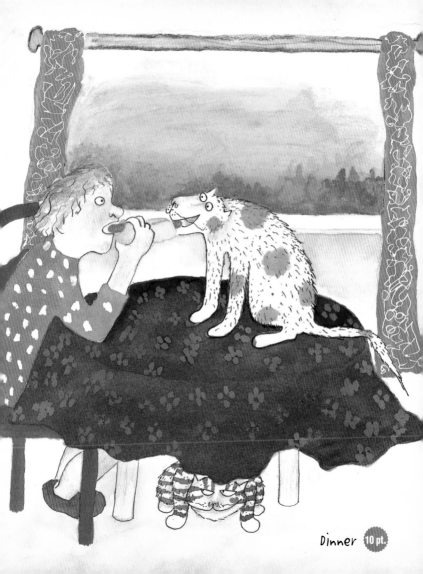

Dinner 10 pt.

STEALING

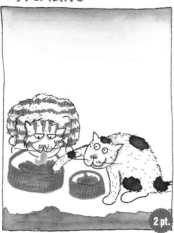

From other cat—dinner

2 pt.

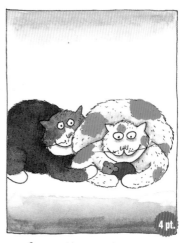

From other cat—prey

4 pt.

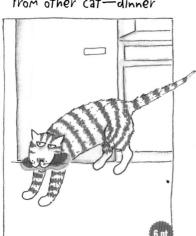

From kitchen

6 pt.

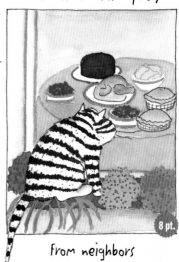

From neighbors

8 pt.

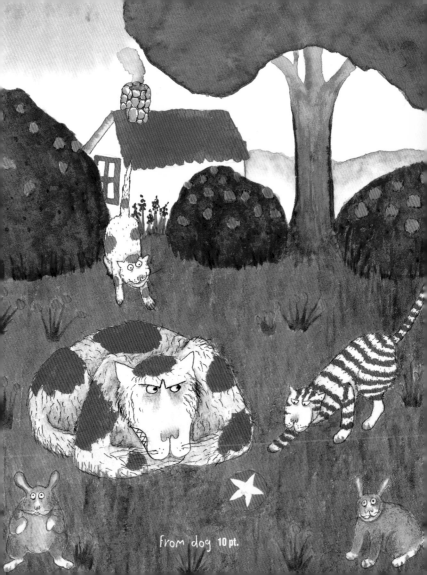

from dog 10 pt.

TRAVELING BY CAR

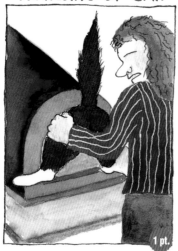

Carrier

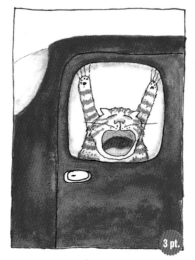

Window

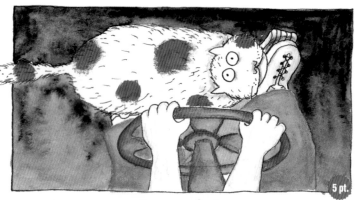

On your feet

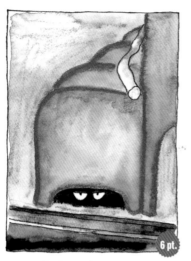

Under the seat

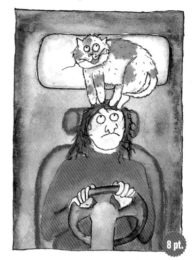

On your head

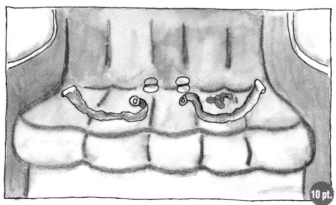

Car accident

USING CATNIP

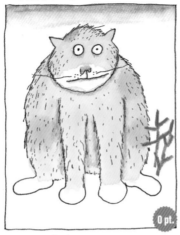

Just says no

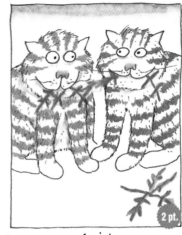

Social

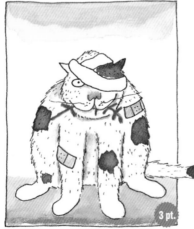

Medicinal

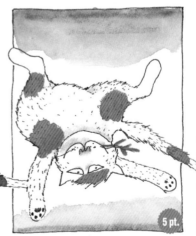

Parties hard

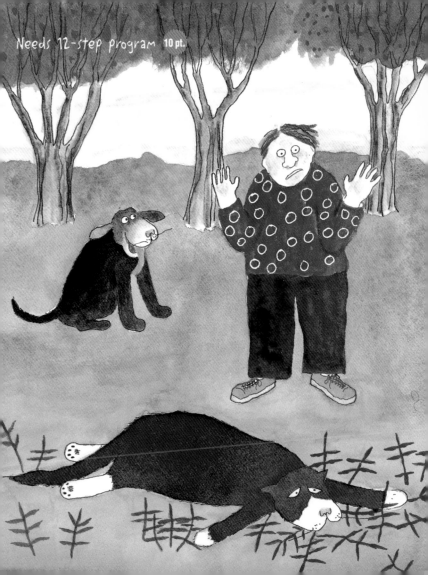

Needs 12-step program 10 pt.

VOCALIZING

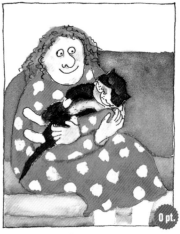

Purrs

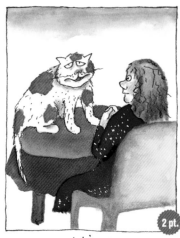

Whines

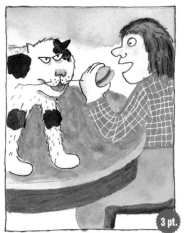

Demands

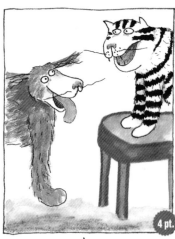

Hisses

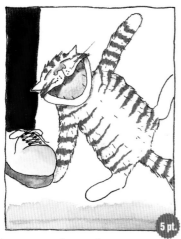

Screeches

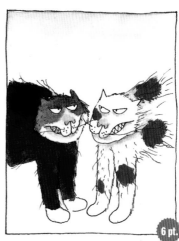

Growls

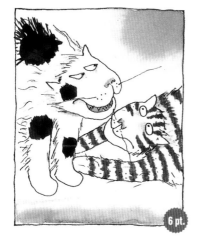

Snarls

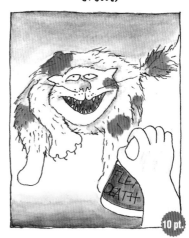

Yowls like fire engine

OTHER WEIRD STUFF

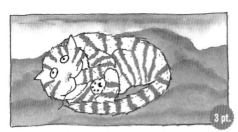

Regressive behavior

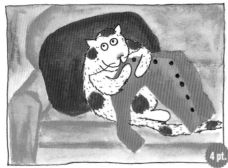

Sucking buttons

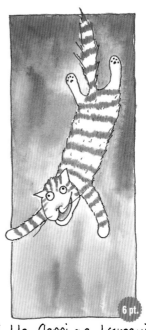

Sudden flapping and screamin

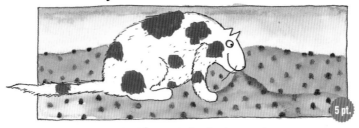

Sucking whole bedspread

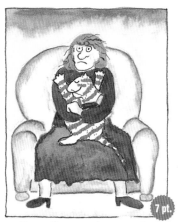

Kneading—ruins costly
new sweater

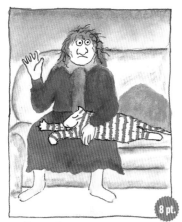

Kneading—shreds last
pair of pantyhose

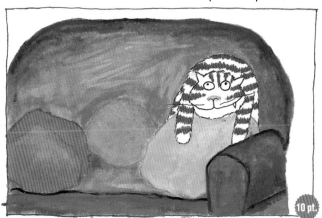

Unwholesome relationship with sofa cushion

KITTY WEIRDNESS SCALE (KWS)

Note: Ranges are not specifically scaled. Some begin at 0, while others "start" at 5. Those that begin at a higher number are considered more weird, but they may not apply to your cat at all. Naturally, in such cases the score is 0.

Score only once in each category of behavior, e.g. eating, personal cleanliness, and so on.

275 points or more: Sorry to have to tell you this, but you have one weird cat (as if you didn't already know)! Clinical studies reveal that cats in this category do best in the wild. Verify that your animal is not a Tasmanian Devil. If this feline is still intact, you are to be congratulated for your forbearance and good will. On the other hand, you may be as crazy as your cat. Some people think this is a compliment.

225 to 274 points: Frisky is OK, but this cat is probably too much to handle. We have tried oral administration of catnip to slow down such hyperactive behavior, but unfortunately we just got an active animal with a substance abuse problem. Behavior modification techniques have been found to be helpful in cases such as these, but it's important to be clear about who is modifying whom! Have your cat send for our booklet *Training Your Human: From Cleanliness to the Can Opener.* Cat owners may send for *Train Your Cat in 10,000 Frustrating Lessons.*

180 to 224 points: What you have here is a playful, active cat who

probably has somewhat of a behavior problem, yet is lots of fun to play with. Kittens and young cats often fall into this category. If you have an older cat who achieves this score, please let us know. The AARF (American Association of Retired Felines) wants this kind of information.

135 to 179 points: There's no other way to say it—your cat is average. Now, we know that no cat is "just average" and we don't want to put pejorative labels on our pets, but when your cat scores right in the middle, there is no way to avoid stating the obvious. If you want your cat to be more unique, you might start by looking at your own behavior. Loosen up a little. Try to show your cat how to have a good time. Helping your cat learn the Macarena may be good therapy for both of you!

90 to 134 points: Some people actually like cats who aren't too weird. That's OK, but as we get toward the inactive part of the KWS, we begin to get into nonfeline territory. You may want to review your cat owner's manual for help in identifying your animal's species. (Gender too, if you don't want several more of the same running around the place.)

45 to 89 points: This animal may be clinically depressed. Perhaps the problem is loneliness. Consider getting another cat or two. Remember, there is no such thing as too many cats, especially if they just lie about like this one. Antidepressant medications may also help, but Prozac has been known to induce suicidal behavior in cats—one actually went out and got a job!

44 points or fewer: Caution—this may not be a cat you are dealing with. Verify that your animal is a) alive b) not a footstool and c) not a stuffed animal. But beware of false identification. After all, remember where the term "catatonic" originated.

ABOUT THE AUTHOR

Missy Dizick is a devoted cat watcher who is inspired by her "five rollicking pussycats," Loulou, Charlie, Bobby, Betty, and Weirdo. Her previous books include the controversial Cats Are Better Than Dogs, preceded by the disloyal Dogs Are Better Than Cats (coauthored with Mary Bly), which she is still trying to live down. Her prize-winning artwork appears on calendars and note cards and has been exhibited in galleries and museums in California and New York.

Ms. Dizick resides in Napa, California, where she has an absolutely smashing garden.

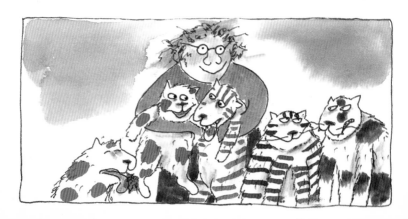